KEEPING A CLEAN HEART

IN A DIRTY WORLD

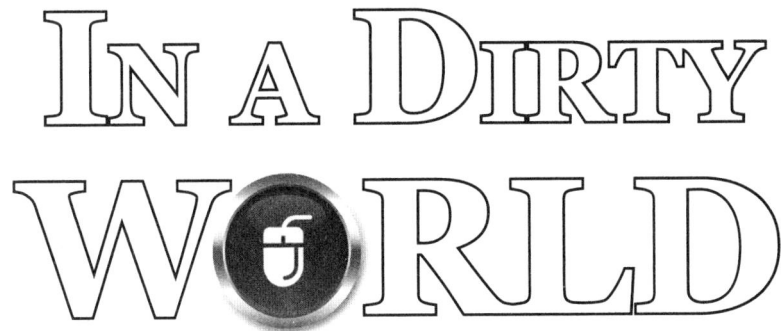

A "G" RATED ANSWER TO AN "X" RATED PROBLEM

Keeping a Clean Heart in a Dirty World

ISBN 978-0-943593-91-3
Copyright © 2012 Peter Enns
Tulsa, OK 74133

www.mycleanheart.com

www.goodwordinternational.com

Cover Design: Markus Pilsl

Text Design Consultant: Lisa Simpson
www.simpsonproductions.net

All Scriptures are from the KJV and NKJV Bible

Dedication & Acknowledgements

This book is dedicated to families who desire to serve the LORD. Joshua was 110 years of age when he said, *"As for me and my house we will serve the LORD."*

Most likely he was a grandfather and we want to include grandparents, who like Joshua, are praying for their extended families, in this dedication.

Secondly this book is dedicated to families who still have children living at home. With all the outside influences that affect our lives today, raising Godly children takes more than the Wisdom of Solomon. But we serve One who is greater than Solomon was; His name is Jesus.

A note of thanks is in order to all those individuals who have helped make the writing of this book possible. Thanks to Dorothy, my wife who encouraged me to write a book on this most difficult subject.

To Brenda Chapman, our oldest daughter and the mother of three. She called me and gave me a renewed awareness of the challenges today's kids have to face.

To our daughter Kimberly Thomas, for her hours of proof reading, as well as providing her professional input as a licensed Marriage and Family Therapist.

A word of appreciation is in order to Renée Gilligan, for her help in editing the original manuscript for this book.

Statement of Purpose
Keeping A Clean Heart In A Dirty World!

Sexual temptation is as old as the human race! Now porn on the internet and on other digital devices is turning pornography into a worldwide epidemic.

Addressing the exploding problem of internet porn, in an online open letter to churches, Dr. Chuck Swindoll, the radio host on **Insight for Living** says:

"The most recent studies available suggest that one out of every two people - that's 50% of those sitting in our church pews, are looking at and/or could be addicted to Internet pornography."

As alarming as it is, just talking about the problem will never solve it. There is an answer! It's in the Bible and it includes, **The Clean Heart Prayer!**

The Biblical story of King David and Bathsheba and the parable of the Prodigal Son are examples of decent people who got caught up doing bad things.

In spite of human weakness and moral failures, David is a testimony of someone who was able to make a comeback to lead a useful and productive life. So can anyone else willing to follow his example.

The Clean Heart Prayer will work for anyone!

Contents

Introduction

A "G" Rated Answer to an "X" Rated Problem!

"I am the way, the truth and the life." These words spoken by Jesus, in John 14:6, answer the age old question; "What is Truth?"

Again quoting Jesus, in John 8:32 He said, *"You shall know the truth and the truth shall set you free."*

The truth is: "We are living in a dirty world."

Psalm 119:9, likely written by the psalmist David, asks the question: *"How can a young man cleanse his way?"* The answer; *"By taking heed according to Your word."*

Following the Last Supper, and what we might call a Communion Service, Jesus prayed a prayer to God for His disciples. Then in His closing statement, he included the entire world in that prayer:

"I do not pray that You should take them out of the world, but that You should keep them from the evil one. They are not of the world, just as I am not of the world. Sanctify them by Your truth. Your Word is truth."

Keeping a Clean Heart in a Dirty World will help answer the prayer of Jesus, in your personal life. After you read this book, please get additional copies to share with your family and friends.

THE CLEAN HEART PRAYER

"Create in me a clean heart, O God; and renew a right spirit within me." (Psalm 51:10)

"Let the words of my mouth, and the meditation of my heart, be acceptable in thy sight, O Lord". (Psalm 19:14)

"Thy word have I hid in mine heart, that I might not sin against thee." (Psalm 119:11)

"I will walk within my house with a perfect heart. I will set no wicked thing before mine eyes;" (Psalm. 101:2-3)

"As for me and my house, we will serve the Lord." (Joshua 24:15)

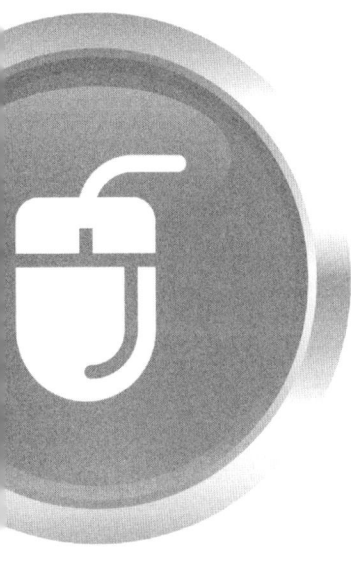

The Preamble

The Players

David and Bathsheba
An Opportunist Finding
An Opportunity

The Pleasure

Begins in the Eyes
Numbs Good Judgment
Is Not Satisfied Until it is too Late

The Price

Murder
A Broken Home
Loss of Reputation

The Penalty

The Death of a Baby
The Loss of Friendship
A King in Disgrace

The Prayer

Acknowledge – Confess – Repent
Ask God to Do What Only He Can Do
Forgive – Create – Restore

The Prodigal

Caught by a Thought
Dreamer to Schemer
The Right to be Wrong

The Pull

Leaving the Farm
What's the Harm
Fooled by Charm

The Pigpen

Cash to Burn
Lessons to Learn
Time to Turn

11

The Power

Want Power
Will Power
Word Power

The Party

New Robe
New Shoes
New Ring

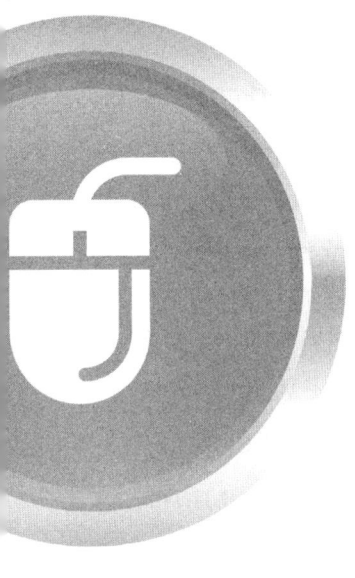

Setting the Stage

THE ROYAL AFFAIR

She was taking a bath where King David could see,
From the roof of his house, just like watching TV.
Seeing her there was a beautiful sight,
And David decided, "I want her tonight!"

Bathsheba said ,"Yes." She could have said, "No."
Her husband was gone and no one would know.
Bathsheba knew she was breaking her vow,
But gave in to the king who wanted her now.

As she left the king's bed, they both were aware,
That they had sinned when they had the affair.
It had felt good, but now they felt bad.
Bathsheba was pregnant, and he was the dad.

To cover his sin, here was his plan.
"I'll bring home Uriah, as fast as I can.
He'll sleep with Bathsheba, and he will believe,
It was his seed that made her conceive."

But Uriah said, "No, I'll sleep on the floor,"
Taking his roll, he slept by the door.
"My men are in battle, fighting out there.
To sleep with my wife, just wouldn't be fair."

When the plan failed, King David said, "Fine,
I'll throw a party and he'll drink my wine.
He'll forget about war and his passions will stir.
When he goes to bed, he'll be sleeping with her."

But again he said, "No!" This was David's last try.
To hide the affair, Uriah must die!
David was willing to take his friend's life,
To hide the affair that he had with his wife.

God was displeased with what David had done,
Causing the death of Bathsheba's new son.
One night with Bathsheba! He'd made a bad trade.
Murder and death was the price that he paid.

© Peter Enns 2011

Nightfall had come over the royal city of Jerusalem. The King had already retired for the night but he could not fall asleep. Leaving his bedroom, he walked out onto the balcony of the palace. As King David stood there peering into the darkness, he saw an alluring sight that caught his attention.

In the distance, he could see the image of a woman. She was taking a bath and she was beautiful. Observing her body as she moved in the light was a breathtaking scene for the King to see. Forgetting about sleep, now he was wide awake.

Was this the first time King David had encountered this situation? Could it be that he had been on this balcony before on other sleepless nights with anticipation of what he might see?

Was it possible that the wicked one, the enemy of David's soul was setting up a trap that would ultimately ensnare David? In any event, David was captivated by what his eyes saw as he continued to gaze at this stunning woman.

Like someone watching the preview of a movie, he made the decision to stay for the main feature. Rather than turning away and saying, *"No,"* to sexual temptation and lust, King David allowed his passions to be stirred. "No one else was watching him, or knew what he was doing. Why not look?" David thought to himself.

What had started as just a thought in David's imaginative mind suddenly became an idea. He liked what he had seen and could not get her off his mind. Why not find out who this woman was? Maybe he could meet her. Perhaps she could even become his wife.

According to the custom of the day, multiple wives were a common and accepted practice. If this woman was not married, he might well be able to take her as his legal marriage partner. To find out more about her, the king ordered a background check.

When David got back the report that he had asked for, he discovered she was already married to another man. This should have been enough information for David to make the right decision. Just knowing that she already was someone else's wife told him she was definitely off limits to him.

He discovered that her name was Bathsheba. She was the daughter of Eliam, and Uriah was her husband. Uriah was in military service and currently, he was away from home. The scriptures indicate that Bathsheba had just finished her monthly menstrual cycle, so obviously she was not pregnant.

Something had started happening in David's mind that he was enjoying. It was a spirit of lust at work in his thought life. By willfully entertaining passionate thoughts, David had opened the door and allowed a seductive spirit to enter into his mind and his imagination.

Why was this woman taking a bath where her naked body was so visible and on display? Did she have an ulterior motive in her behavior?

Was Bathsheba the enticing bait the enemy was trying to use to destroy David, a man after God's own heart? Was she an opportunist looking for an opportunity?

Being home alone as a wife, she may have had sexual desires that were not being satisfied. When an invitation from King David was delivered to Bathsheba to join him at the palace, the stage was set.

How could she refuse an audience with the most powerful man in the kingdom? As inviting as it was, she still had the right to say, *"No."* That night, David and Bathsheba entered into an immoral sexual relationship.

What a price they both would have to pay for their decision. Before it was all over, there would be the murder of an honorable husband, a broken home and finally the death of an innocent baby.

There would also be other serious consequences that would haunt the king for the rest of his life.

From the loss of his reputation, to a negative influence from his children, the penalty of David's immoral actions would leave a permanent mark on his life and affect the very effectiveness as the King of Israel.

The reason this sordid story is in the Scriptures is so we can learn some powerful and important lessons from the experiences of King David and Bathsheba.

It shows us the power of temptation and also demonstrates God's love and mercy and the grace of forgiveness and the path to restoration.

The fact that after all this, God still called David a man after his own heart and continued to bless him, should be an encouragement to everyone.

Like David, when we acknowledge our wrong doing and ask for God's help, we can be restored and once again live the life of an overcomer.

19

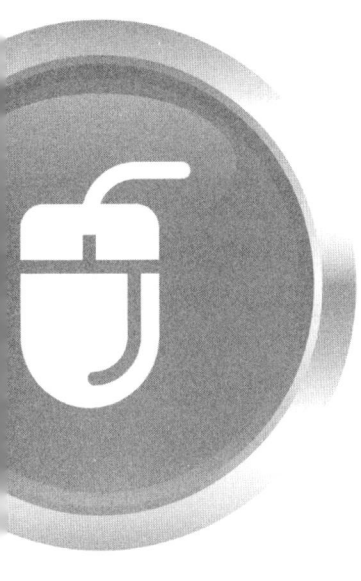

David,

a Man after God's

Own Heart

THE BATTLE IS THE LORD'S!

For forty days, morning and night,
King Saul had watched the news.
Goliath was the anchorman,
Who shared his worldly views.

Saul believed his boasting words.
He marveled at his size.
Goliath's shield and flashing sword,
Put fear in King Saul's eyes.

But David knew what God had said.
A boy, still in his youth,
He wasn't moved by what he saw.
To him, God's Word was truth.

God had said, "Don't be afraid,
I'll win the fight for you."
Just like the lion and the bear,
He killed that giant too.

When life's giants cross your path,
Don't listen to their views.
Change channels! Turn from doubt to faith.
You have the right to choose.

© Peter Enns 2011

22

David had a passion! Already as a teenaged lad, he had encountered physical dangers that would have stopped most grown men. The youngest of Jesse's family clan, David had seven older brothers. While his brothers carried out their military duties as soldiers in King Saul's army, David spent his time as a shepherd, watching over and feeding his father's flocks of sheep.

David would never forget that most fateful day when he was summoned to come back to the house. Samuel, a well-known prophet of God was there and he had asked to see David. The prophet Samuel had come to deliver a very important message from God Almighty.

The LORD had told the prophet to go and anoint one of the sons of Jesse to be the next King of Israel. One by one, each of his older brothers had been rejected for this high position. David was the only son remaining, so this had to be God's choice. Even though he was very young, when Samuel saw David, he knew this was the one God had chosen as the future king.

Taking the horn of anointing oil he had brought, Samuel poured the oil on David's head. To others watching, it might have looked as if David was chosen for this high position by default. But both Samuel and David knew that he was God's choice. In his heart, David had the strong assurance that God had a special plan for his life and that he was called for a definite purpose.

For David, there were no immediate changes. Each day he still went back to the menial task of being a shepherd.

Spending long hours alone on the hillside gave David the opportunity to develop an intimate and uninterrupted relationship with God. To David, God was just like a loving shepherd who was taking care of his young sheep.

As a shepherd, there were slow and boring days but there were also some days of great excitement. Keeping away the intruders who would try to steal his sheep, David was being prepared for a special assignment. Facing the wild animals with just a sling in his hand, David was becoming a skilled marksman.

David took his life as a shepherd very seriously. On several occasions, he had risked his very life for the safety of the sheep. When a ferocious bear came and tried to steal a small lamb, David killed the bear with just his bare hands.

On another occasion, a fierce lion attacked and once again David came out victorious. David knew this was more than just human courage and skill. It was God who was helping him fight and protect his sheep from these wild and dangerous animals.

King Saul, who was Israel's first king, had started out well. The scriptures say that in the beginning, Saul was small in his own eyes. But as time went by, things began to change. Rather than doing what God was telling him to do, Saul became arrogant and walked in disobedience.

His days as King of Israel were now numbered. Although Saul did not know it, eventually God was going to give the kingdom to David. It was during this time period that the nation of Israel came under hostile attack.

The formidable Philistine army along with their champion, the giant Goliath, came and challenged Israel to do battle. In all of King Saul's army there was no one willing to fight this champion. It was certainly understandable, because Goliath literally was a giant of a man.

Standing better than nine feet tall, this huge giant was an intimidating sight. He was skilled in combat and he knew no defeat. With his heavy armor, full length shield and sharp spear, Goliath was the equivalent of a human tank. It was plain to see there was no one in Saul's army who was equal to Goliath, either in size or in the ability to fight in hand to hand combat.

News traveled slowly in those days. With his sons in the military, Jesse had a vested interest in the war. He wanted to know first hand, what was going on in the battle against the Philistines.

One day Jesse asked his son David to leave the sheep, go to the battlefield and bring back a report of what was happening. Loaded with food and refreshments for his brothers, David made his way to the valley where the soldiers were camped.

While David was still talking to his brothers, suddenly the air was split by the blood curdling scream of Goliath, the champion of the Philistines. He didn't know it, but life was about to change for David.

For forty days Goliath had been challenging the army of King Saul to send someone out to come and fight with him. Perhaps humiliated and somewhat embarrassed, David's brothers told him to leave the dangerous battle scene and return home to his duties as a shepherd.

But something was stirring in David's heart. Since he believed that one day he would become the King of Israel, David knew that God had a way to remove this mountain of a man who was cursing God and threatening the very survival of Saul's kingdom.

As he lingered on the scene, David became aware that there was a reward offered to anyone willing to go and do battle with Goliath. The word was out that King Saul was offering great riches, no family property taxes and even the king's daughter in marriage to the man who would take on and defeat the giant. Among all the soldiers, there was no one willing to take the offer.

David continued to talk to the different soldiers in the army. The king's offered reward began to intrigue him. While everyone else including the king seemed to be terrified, something was happening to David. Faith was rising up in his heart. To David it was no longer the Philistines fighting the Israelites. It was a battle of evil against God Almighty!

While the other soldiers in Saul's army kept talking fear and doubt, David was speaking faith. He talked about fighting both a bear and a lion, and how God had delivered him from danger.

David's positive words penetrated the atmosphere like a beam of light in a dark night. It wasn't long before the stories David was telling were reported to King Saul. Saul may not have recognized it, but there was an anointing from God on David's life. His supernatural experiences as a shepherd boy defending the flock of sheep had prepared him for this day.

David told the king that the battle was not his to win but it was the LORD's battle. Then with a divine burst of enthusiasm, David volunteered to go and fight Goliath.

Defying all human logic, King Saul agreed to let him go. Not trained in military combat, David felt uncomfortable wearing the armor of a soldier, so instead he chose only the weapons he had used as a shepherd. Armed with only a sling and five smooth stones, the young man stepped out to meet his foe.

27

As this giant of a man, Goliath, was approaching, David ran to meet him. The words out of David's mouth were words of faith as he declared, *"I come to you in the Name of my God!"* The exciting story of David, the shepherd, defeating Goliath, the giant, has become an all time legend, inspiring people to succeed against all odds.

After his dramatic victory, David's life was in for a drastic change! At King Saul's invitation, David went to live at the palace. He was extolled and honored as a hero by everyone, including the King. It must have been a high moment in his life as the young women began to sing and chant the praises about David, the Giant killer.

Something was happening that would soon alter and put an end to his new found lifestyle. As the public show of affection for David increased, it quickly became evident that the people were honoring David above King Saul. Being a proud man, the accolades offered to David became offensive to King Saul.

It wasn't long until a spirit of jealousy entered the king's heart. He now felt threatened by David and began to hate him. On several different occasions, in a hot fit of rage, Saul threw his spear at David, but each time he missed his target. God was protecting David because He had a plan for him that no one could destroy.

When Saul had been anointed as the first King of Israel, he had no example to follow. The only models of kings and kingdoms Saul knew about were the ungodly nations that surrounded Israel. This is why the spiritual role of the prophets in Israel had become so important.

God would give His message to the prophet, who in turn would deliver His message to the king. It was then up to the king to follow God's instructions. Not listening to the prophet would ultimately cost King Saul both his position and his life.

In the beginning, Saul had seen himself small in his own eyes. Drunk on power and prestige, his concept had changed. He was the king and chose to do things his own way. What David may not have known, was that because of Saul's disobedience to the word of the prophet, the Spirit of the LORD had already departed from King Saul.

Now feelings of depression and hopelessness were haunting the king. At those moments, he would call for David who was a skilled musician. As David played the harp, the sound of his anointed music filled the room and it drove out the spirit of anger, fear and despair and calmed King Saul's tormented mind for awhile.

Watching King Saul, David knew it was time to leave his comfortable new surroundings. The king seemed to be losing his mind and for his own safety, David needed to get away. Possibly, King Saul had heard about the prophet Samuel going to anoint David as the future king.

Instead of a military hero, David was now a threat to King Saul and he had to get rid of him. Instead of asking God what to do, King Saul was led by his own suspicious mind. No longer on speaking terms with Samuel, what else could he do?

A providential thing happened to David while he was still living in the palace. King Saul had a son named Jonathon. A great friendship began to develop between the shepherd and the prince. Becoming best of friends, they entered into a special covenant relationship they would honor for the rest of their lives.

Strange as it may seem, when he left the palace, David did not return home to his father's house. It may have been the jealousy of his own brothers that kept him away. They were older and more experienced and maybe unwilling to accept or believe that David had been chosen as a future king.

Perhaps he stayed away for his own safety. Obviously if King Saul was out to kill him, David's home would be a likely place to look for him. Instead, David went and hid in caves. Having lived the rugged life of a shepherd, he knew how to take care of himself without needing any of the luxury and comforts of his father's house.

The next ten years of David's life seemed like a blur. Constantly on the run, he was trying to avoid King Saul, who by now was obsessed with destroying his life. David had a small group of loyalists with him, but he knew they were no match for Saul's entire army.

David had opportunity after opportunity to kill King Saul, but each time he refused. David had made the decision to trust God for His protection. When close friends suggested that these were God-given opportunities, David refused to accept their counsel.

Because Samuel had also anointed Saul as the king, David refused to touch God's anointed man. To David, the anointing of God was a serious and supernatural thing. He was willing to wait on God's timing rather than to take things into his own hands and make them happen by his own efforts.

One of David's more dramatic experiences happened in one of the caves where he was hiding. While in hot pursuit of David, King Saul and his army stopped at the mouth of the cave so he could attend to personal matters. Turning the cave into his private men's room, King Saul was unaware of David's presence in the cave.

Seeing the king in a crouched and compromising position, David crept up behind him. Taking his sword, David cut off a piece of King Saul's royal garment. Here was solid evidence of his good will toward the king. At that very moment, David could easily have destroyed King Saul, but once again he chose not to do so.

It was during his hard experiences as a fugitive that David wrote many of the great Psalms. While some of his writings may sound like a country songwriter, singing the blues, they always end with a note of victory. David was confident that ultimately God would vindicate and deliver him from his troubles.

Certainly, thoughts of, *"Why is God allowing this to happen to me?"* Must have crossed David's mind. There was no question that David had experienced a mighty victory against the giant Goliath. If God was on his side, why were all these bad things still happening to him?

David never seemed to have lacked courage but he was still in the learning process of becoming a leader. More than just being brave, leadership also required that he have wisdom and understanding. David was finding out that some of the most important lessons in life come through difficult experiences.

Still a young man, David was in his late twenties when King Saul's rule was coming to a bitter end. As King Saul led his army into a heated battle, both the king and his son, Jonathan, were mortally wounded. Aware that his life was over, King Saul fell on his own sword and died.

With the death of King Saul, the time had come for David to be crowned as the next King of Israel. He was facing the task of establishing his kingdom and fulfilling his God-appointed purpose. At the age of just thirty, David was beginning a reign that would last forty years.

As the King of Israel, David had absolute power. There were no other elected officials and everyone else was appointed by him. In this form of government, there were no checks and balances. With this absolute power also came absolute responsibility. If things did not go well in the kingdom, there was no one else to blame.

It was customary for a king to go into battle with his army. The king was also the military leader and it was his role to make the strategic decisions. No one had more to gain or lose than the king. Losing the battle could mean losing the kingdom and likely losing his own life.

Everything was going great in David's life. He was a good king and was well liked by the people. There was a relative calm in his kingdom with only small military skirmishes. While he had soldiers away from home and on assigned duty, there were no major battles going on.

It was time for David to take a break and enjoy the benefits of being King of Israel. In his past, David had fought a bear, a lion and even a giant.

He had also overcome several attempts on his life. Now he was about to face an enemy he had never faced before. In this setting is where the encounter between David and Bathsheba takes place.

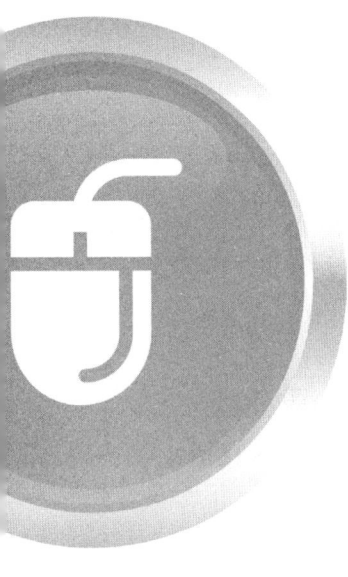

Bathsheba,

a Bathing Beauty

WOMAN

A beautiful being. Adam's surprise!
She put love in his heart and a thrill in his eyes.
God knew what he needed; He gave him the best.
Husband and wife; His first couple was blessed.

Fulfilling his needs, by God's design!
With his first look, Adam said, "She is mine."
A wondrous creation, inside and out.
She understood what she was about.

By the look in her eyes, she had a way,
Of letting him know what she wanted to say.
Pleasing and pleasure went hand in hand.
She got what she wanted without a demand.

A lover, a mother, a mate and a friend.
Her gift to her husband was love without end.
Matched for each other, as woman and man.
A living example of God's perfect plan.

© Peter Enns 2011

Bathsheba was a woman. That alone made her a unique being. There has always been a mystique about a woman that no man has ever been able to fully understand or explain.

By her look, her walk and the sound of her voice, woman, by design, has been attractive to the opposite sex. Her appearance on the scene commands attention.

Both Adam and Eve had been created in God's image. He was created from the dust of the earth and she was created from a rib that God had taken from Adam's side. They possessed wonderful creative power and abilities.

As man and woman, they were God's masterpiece of creation. Woman was blessed with a tender and compassionate heart. What better demonstrates God's loving care for us, than a mother's love for her child?

As a parallel to her compassion, woman was also endowed with a longing for romance; with a need to be needed, and a desire to be appreciated.

Her presence brings warmth and elegance into the atmosphere. With her gentle spirit, she can penetrate the heart of even the toughest man.

Something else that no man has ever fully understood is a woman's intuitiveness and discernment. It is as though she feels or knows something she cannot put into words.

Beyond human logic, she is able to recognize the real purpose or the motive behind seemingly harmless acts or words. She knows what she knows, but can't tell you why.

Like everything else God has created, the influence and charm of a woman can be used positively or negatively. She can use her gifting to bless and heal as well as to hurt and destroy.

Throughout the pages of history (including current news headlines), there are stories of powerful and intelligent men who have succumbed to the temptation of subtle and seductive women.

In our story, Bathsheba found herself the object of David's desire and passion. The decision she was about to make and what she would allow to happen would change her life and the life of her family forever. While David was the instigator, Bathsheba became a willing partner.

In the eyes of most men, there is nothing more beautiful than a woman. From her hair to her eyes; from her lips to the contour of the rest of her body, her male counterpart is fascinated by her physical beauty.

A woman can use this charm and power for good or for evil. Beauty is in the eyes of the beholder. God in His infinite wisdom, placed within the male, the ability and the desire to appreciate this beautiful physical work of art. It was a created masterpiece made from the rib of the first man.

"Wow!" May well have been the first word Adam uttered when he awoke and took a look at the woman, God had created for him.

As a young man, David had already showed an interest in the opposite sex. Getting Saul's daughter as a prize for killing the giant had been part of his motivation.

Now as a middle aged man, David was still motivated by the same thing. Having seen Bathsheba, he wanted to be with her and nothing could stop him.

In the narrative of this story in the scriptures, it simply states that Bathsheba was beautiful. Likely she was aware of her own good looks and David's expressed appreciation of her physical charm may have added to here willingness to meet this powerful man.

In today's language, a beautiful woman is often referred to as having a perfect body. From God's perspective, true beauty begins on the inside. It is in the heart that the real beauty of a woman resides.

There is no word that better describes perfection than the word "Love." There is also no more destructive word than the word "Lust."

Ultimately, it was lust and not love that drew Bathsheba from her home and into the privacy of King David's palatial bedroom.

Bathsheba was married to Uriah, a Hittite, a man of the Jewish faith. (His name means YHWH is my light).

Being his wife, she most likely was of the same belief. As a soldier in David's army, Uriah was away from home and on military duty at this time.

Bathsheba must have known of the religious and moral law of her faith. The marriage covenant required her to be faithful to her husband even in his absence.

After all, he was probably missing her too. As we will see later, Uriah was a man of discipline who was well able to control his passions.

Having experienced male companionship, as a young wife home alone, she may have missed the affection of her husband away on military duty.

For whatever reason, the scriptures tell us she had just completed her menstrual cycle, indicating that at this time she was not pregnant.

What would cause a young and attractive wife of a soldier, serving in the army to be willing to break her marriage vows? Was it flattering words coming from the lips of a powerful King?

Was it her desire for sexual fulfillment? Was it a spirit of lust that was tempting Bathsheba to be unfaithful? It may well have been a combination of all of these things.

Was Bathsheba taking a bath in an inappropriate location? Did she know she was being watched? These are details we will never know. What we do know, is that one day there was a knock on her door.

Standing in front of her was someone with a royal invitation. She was being invited to have an audience with King David. What did the king want with her? What could she have to offer him?

Whatever it was, she was soon going to find out. Gracious compliments, valuable gifts, and the elegant palace likely all contributed to the bad decision Bathsheba made that night. She said, "Yes," to David's invitation, when she should have said, "No."

As King David reached out to touch her, what would happen next was her's to decide. The pull of sexual temptation was strong! He was a powerful man and she was a beautiful woman. Now they were alone together.

Overcome by the passion and pleasure of the moment, the consequences of their behavior may not have been in their minds. Lust has a way of dulling the conscience.

King David and Bathsheba would both soon discover the horrendous price they would have to pay for their illicit sexual behavior.

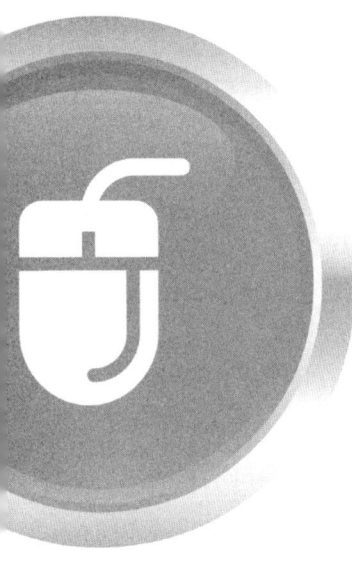

The Spirit of Lust

Sex was God's Idea!

God Created it to be a Delightful Experience Between a Husband and Wife

The sexual experience between a man and a woman, within the God ordained confines of marriage is beautiful and fulfilling. It is a gift from God to mankind. Were it not for sexual pleasure in marriage, most likely the pain of childbirth would have stopped the human procreative process.

God, who is all wise, included the pleasure of having a sexual relationship as part of the human experience in marriage. Sexual pleasures may be momentary and fleeting but the reward of bringing children into this world lives on forever. As an added bonus, it seems that God also intended sexual pleasure to be a bonding force between husband and wife.

Psychiatrists and psychologists describe the mind as the biggest human sex organ, with the eye being the gateway to the mind. This is where sexual ideas first develop. Here is the process: what first begins as a thought turns into an idea; the idea creates desire; desire develops into a plan; and the plan turns into the desired action.

Because we are more than a mind and a body, there are also evil spiritual forces that can influence human sexual behavior. Evil wants to pervert God's intended purpose for sex. Bizarre sexual conduct makes this evident. God's intent for sex was to be an experience of grace and beauty between a husband and wife.

Admire!

Admiring someone of the opposite sex is as natural as the air we breathe or the water we drink. It is like two magnets that are attracted to each other by an unseen force. God Himself, placed this function in the makeup of both man and woman.

Desire!

Admire can quickly turn into desire. Nowhere do we see a better illustration of strong sexual desire than we do in the animal kingdom.

Here, two males will often fight each other to the point of permanent injury or even death for the opportunity of sexual fulfillment and gratification. All logic and reason seems to have been abandoned and no price is too high.

With both testosterone and adrenaline surging in the body, the undisciplined human can act the same way. Logic goes out of the window and morals are easily forgotten.

However, humans differ from all the rest of God's creation. They have a mind to think and the will to choose. For that reason, sexual desires between a man and a woman have to be kept within predetermined limits.

Out of control sexual desires have destroyed kingdoms and empires. Still today, unchecked desire is destroying careers, businesses, churches and the most hurtful of all, it is breaking up marriages and families.

Sexual desire is God's gift to mankind, but it must be kept under control. As a guide, God has given humans a code of conduct found in the scriptures. Hebrews 13:4 says *"Marriage is honorable in all and the bed undefiled; but whoremongers and adulterers God will judge."*

Require!

When "Desire, out of control," takes over, what is right or wrong, as well as the consequence of the behavior, is easily overridden. Desire says, "This is what I now require. I cannot be happy or satisfied without it. I will do whatever it takes to get it."

Acquire

Acquire completes the cycle of "Desire, out of control." Desire says, "I will make it mine. I will demand it, command it, and brand it as my own. If it belongs to someone else, I will buy it. If I can't buy it, I will steal it."

Fire!

The result of "Desire out of control," is like a burning fire. Fire is called a good servant but a bad master. For that reason it has to be kept under control. Strange as it may

44

seem, Solomon, the son of David and Bathsheba, wrote these words.

Proverbs 6:27 - 29: *"Can a man take fire to his bosom, and his clothes not be burned? Can one walk on hot coals, and his feet not be seared?" "So is he who goes in to his neighbor's wife; whoever touches her shall not be innocent."*

When Desire Becomes Lust

There is more to life than what is experienced by what we see, hear, smell, taste or feel. When we say, "It doesn't make sense," What we really are saying is that something cannot be defined or explained through the five natural human senses.

Having a "sixth sense" is a common term used to describe intuition or discernment. Beyond the ability of the mind, there are also spiritual forces at work in our world.

There is an unseen source of good as well as an unseen source of evil. We understand that God is the source of all good and the source of all evil is the Devil.

The life of Jesus on this earth demonstrated the goodness of God. Jesus also confirmed that the Devil is evil.

In John 10:10, He said, "The thief does not come except to steal, and to kill, and to destroy. I have come that they may have life, and that they may have it more abundantly."

The scriptures teach that there are angels from God sent to earth to watch over and protect human life. Likewise, the scriptures also tell us there are evil forces at work in the affairs of humans.

They seek to influence and control human behavior negatively. It may well be that there are actual evil lusting spirit beings who have the assignment of causing moral human corruption. Could it be that the evil lure of pornography and immoral temptation is a direct assault of the wicked one on humanity?

Human beings have a free will and have the choice of who and what will influence their behavior. The scriptures have many insightful and helpful instructions on how to deal with evil temptation.

When Jesus, the Son of God, was tempted by the evil one, He set the example. His defense to every temptation was, *"It is written,"* followed by a quotation of the scriptures from the Old Testament.

Human decisions are based on input and information received and processed by the mind. If the mind is not controlled, it will result in an uncontrolled life.

No normal human being is ever exempt from temptation, and especially from sexual temptation. This fact has been demonstrated over and over again. All too frequently, the TV news headlines lead with stories of lurid behavior.

Lust Numbs Logic and Sound Reasoning

Read the history of great military leaders, presidents and politicians, as well as others in high and powerful positions and the pull of lust quickly becomes evident.

Even among church leadership we have seen individuals robbed of their sound reasoning by uncontrolled sexual appetites. With a numbed conscience, good lives have ended up as moral failures and ruined ministries.

In the book of Proverbs, Solomon gives us a description of a seductive woman trying to entice a young man into having an illicit sexual relationship with her.

Beginning in Proverbs 7:19, here is what it says:

47

> *19 "For my husband is not at home;*
> *He has gone on a long journey;*
> *20 He has taken a bag of money with him,*
> *And will come home on the appointed day."*
> *21 With her enticing speech she caused him to yield,*
> *With her flattering lips she seduced him.*
> *22 Immediately he went after her, as an ox goes to the*
> *slaughter, Or as a fool to the correction of the stocks,*
> *23 Till an arrow struck his liver. As a bird hastens*
> *to the snare, He did not know it would cost his life.*

While this scripture is descriptive of an immoral and seductive woman, certainly it is just as applicable to the actions of a flirtatious man.

The Price of Lust for David and Bathsheba

The passion had subsided and the night had passed, now it was time for Bathsheba to return home. The scriptures are silent as to whether there was any further contact between David and Bathsheba but after about forty five days, she had to get a message to the king.

Her message to the king was, *"I am pregnant with your child."* David was a man with a good name. He was looked up to and admired as a man of God. How could he now save face from what he and Bathsheba had done?

We cannot be certain, but Bathsheba may have been in on the scheme that David concocted. After all, her life and his reputation were at stake as well.

Here was an idea that would surely solve their problem. On the surface, it seemed like it could work, so David began to implement a very wicked plan.

Since Uriah, the soldier and husband of Bathsheba had been away for awhile, why not let him come home? Every soldier in the military deserved a break. Give him some time off for a military furlough.

Having Uriah back home could solve the problem. He had been gone from Bathsheba for an extended period of time, so his passion for her would be high and he and his wife would have sexual relations.

This natural process would produce a pregnancy and Uriah would think that he was the father. No one else would ever know that it was the seed of David, and not that of Uriah, that had made Bathsheba pregnant.

To help make all this happen, Bathsheba would need to participate in the plot by not telling her husband of the affair she had with the king. When Uriah got home, at the king's request, the plan was put into action.

Elegant food was prepared by the palace and delivered to Uriah's home setting the stage for a delightful night. But when the evening was over, to everyone's surprise, Uriah refused to sleep in his own bed with his wife. How could this possibly happen?

As a military man Uriah had learned discipline. Now he was exercising it to the maximum by refusing to have an intimate relationship with his beautiful wife. Perhaps he was taking discipline to the extreme, but there was no doubt Uriah was in control of his passions.

Uriah's reasoning was simple. Being a soldier, he had comrades who at that very moment were on military duty. In his mind, it would be unfair for him to enjoy sexual pleasures with his wife while other men were engaged in military combat.

Rather than sleep in his own bed with Bathsheba, Uriah took his bed roll, left his house, and slept on the floor by the door of the king's house. As unnatural as Uriah's actions seemed, it was God's idea. God was in the process of revealing what David and Bathsheba had done.

The next morning, when word about Uriah's strange and bizarre behavior got back to the king, he must have been dumbfounded! How could this happen? King David was determined to go on with the cover-up so he came up with another idea.

David planned a party to honor Uriah the soldier for his bravery. At the party, he would serve intoxicating wine to Uriah. When he was drunk, Uriah would forget about war and go home to sleep with his wife.

As the party was being prepared, there must have been plenty of good food. We know there was a good supply of strong drink. King David left nothing to chance; he himself, was at the party.

Everything had to be carried out exactly as he had planned. Again, there was plenty of food and everyone seemed to be having a good time. And yes, Uriah was drinking from the king's wine.

But even under the influence of the alcoholic beverages, Uriah stood by his earlier commitment. He would not enjoy physical sex with his wife while his army buddies were at battle. So once again, he took his bed roll and slept by the door of the king's house.

David was frustrated. Covering his affair with Bathsheba now became his obsession. Since Uriah had refused to sleep with his wife, there was only one alternative. Uriah would have to die! The next morning as Uriah was leaving to go to the battlefield, the king handed him a sealed letter addressed to Joab, the army commander.

In the letter, there were specific instructions. The content was hard to believe. It said that when the soldiers were in the heat of battle, Uriah should be assigned to the most dangerous position. As the enemy army was approaching, all supporting troops were to be withdrawn. Uriah should be left to die in battle without anyone to help him.

As difficult as the assignment was, Commander Joab chose to obey it to the letter. When all the circumstances seemed appropriate, Joab did what David had requested. As the enemy attacked, Uriah was assigned to battle. At the given moment, all the supporting troops fell back leaving Uriah unprotected. Uriah died as planned.

An innocent man had been killed and an obedient army general felt guilty over what he had done. It was all part of the price that was paid because King David cast a lusting look at a woman who was not his wife and a beautiful woman who did not have the will to say no.

To the king, whose conscience already had been severely hardened, the word of Uriah's death must have been good news. He had finally succeeded in covering up what he and Bathsheba had done.

Now no one would ever know, and his good name would not be tarnished, or so he thought. Whether she felt truly sorry or not, Bathsheba spent time mourning the death of Uriah her husband.

Then, what could have been seen as an act of compassion, David took her and she became his legal wife. What followed seemed natural. Bathsheba was pregnant.

Now the new baby would be seen as the product of a legitimate marriage relationship. Finally everything was back under control. Or was it?

2 Samuel 11:27 says, *"The thing that David had done, displeased the LORD."*

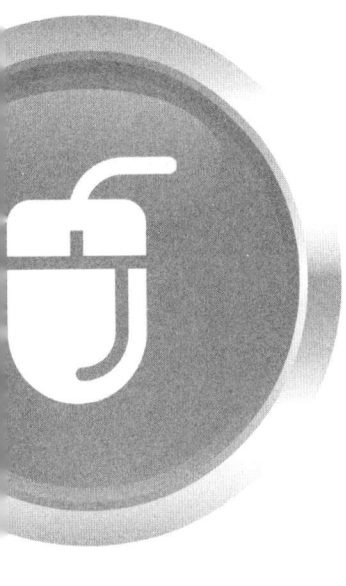

The Prophet

B oth the prophet and the priest were an integral part of the worship structure for Old Testament Jews. The role of the prophet was to deliver God's message to the people. The priest's assignment was to offer animal sacrifices and present the needs of the people to God in worship and prayer.

Other nations had kings and kingdoms that reigned and ruled over their subjects but God wanted to have a direct and personal relationship with His chosen people, the children of Israel. God had written the law with his own finger and He had spoken to Moses face to face.

Here is how God's divine order for his people was structured. God would speak His will and purpose to the prophets and the prophets would in turn communicate God's Word to the fathers.

The father of each household would then instruct and teach the other members in his family what God had said. This required each father to be the spiritual leader of his family.

Watching the other nations who had kings, the leaders of Israel desired to be like them. They refused God's counsel and ultimately God granted their desire. He gave them their first King whose name was Saul.

However, even after the Israelites became a kingdon and had an appointed king, the prophet still played a role in communicating God's messages to the king. A wise king would heed the word of the prophet.

When David became king, as a man after God's own heart, David respected the office of the prophet and wanted to hear what God was saying.

Nathan was one of the prophets of God during the time that David was the king. Supernaturally the Spirit of the LORD revealed to Nathan what had happened in the relationship between David and Bathsheba and in the death of Uriah.

It was one thing for Nathan to know about it, but now the LORD instructed Nathan to go to see King David and confront him about his wrong doing.

In addition, Nathan was to prophesy what would happen both in the near future and the long term as a result of his sinful actions. This was no easy task for the prophet.

It must have taken a lot of boldness on the part of the prophet of God to speak a message of warning or even judgment to the king in the Name of God.

Here is the direct quote of the prophet's message to David from 2 Samuel 12:

> 1) "Then the LORD sent Nathan to David. And he came to him, and said to him: "There were two men in one city, one rich and the other poor.

2) The rich man had exceedingly many flocks and herds."

3) "But the poor man had nothing, except one little ewe lamb which he had bought and nourished; and it grew up together with him and with his children. It ate of his own food and drank from his own cup and lay in his bosom; and it was like a daughter to him.

4) And a traveler came to the rich man, who refused to take from his own flock and from his own herd to prepare one for the wayfaring man who had come to him; but he took the poor man's lamb and prepared it for the man who had come to him."

5) So David's anger was greatly aroused against the man, and he said to Nathan, "As the LORD lives, the man who has done this shall surely die!

6) And he shall restore fourfold for the lamb, because he did this thing and because he had no pity.

7) Then Nathan said to David, "You are the man! Thus says the LORD God of Israel: 'I anointed you king over Israel, and I delivered you from the hand of Saul.

8) I gave you your master's house and your master's wives into your keeping, and gave you the house of Israel and Judah. And if that had been too little, I also would have given you much more!

9) Why have you despised the commandment of the LORD, to do evil in His sight? You have killed Uriah

the Hittite with the sword; you have taken his wife to be your wife, and have killed him with the sword of the people of Ammon.

10) Now therefore, the sword shall never depart from your house, because you have despised Me, and have taken the wife of Uriah the Hittite to be your wife.

11) Thus says the LORD: 'Behold, I will raise up adversity against you from your own house; and I will take your wives before your eyes and give them to your neighbor, and he shall lie with your wives in the sight of this sun.

12) For you did it secretly, but I will do this thing before all Israel, before the sun.

13) So David said to Nathan, "I have sinned against the LORD." And Nathan said to David, "The LORD also has put away your sin; you shall not die.

14) "However, because by this deed you have given great occasion to the enemies of the LORD to blaspheme, the child also who is born to you shall surely die."

15) Then Nathan departed to his house."

Almost immediately things began to unfold, just as the prophet Nathan had prophesied they would.

The baby, who was the product of David's and Bathsheba's illicit relationship, died just a few days after it was born.

David had prayed earnestly, asking for the child to live, but to no avail. Why was God not answering the prayer of David, a man after His own heart? David and Bathsheba were reaping the consequences of their lustful behavior.

Later on when David prayed asking God for forgiveness, God had heard and forgiven him his wrong doing.

The penalty for David's transgression may seem harsh, but so was the pain that he had caused in the lives of others by his irresponsible actions.

Because of his immoral behavior, he had helped breakup a home and a good marriage. David had caused the death of an honorable soldier and forced a general to become a part of his evil scheme.

The result for David and Bathsheba in their illicit affair, had been the death of an innocent baby. But even that was not the end of the repercussion.

Nathan the prophet told David that the sword would never leave his household; meaning that there would be fighting and division amongst his children.

There is a final lesson to be learned from this sad chapter in David's life. When he finally came to his senses; having no where else to go, David confessed his sin. He did not blame Bathsheba or accuse her of trying to seduce him. He accepted responsibility and confessed his sin to God.

Understanding the Heart of David

To understand the heart of David, a good place to look is in the book of Psalms. Two of the most recognized Psalms written by David are Psalm 23 and Psalm 51.

Psalm 23 was likely written by David when he was still a young shepherd boy taking care of the sheep. In spite of David's failure and shortcoming, God still called him *"A man after His own heart."*

Psalm 23

*1) The L*ord *is my shepherd; I shall not want.*

2) He makes me to lie down in green pastures: He leads me beside the still waters.

3) He restores my soul: He leads me in the paths of righteousness for His name's sake.

4) Yea, though I walk through the valley of the shadow of death, I will fear no evil: for You are with me; your rod and your staff they comfort me.

5) You prepare a table before me in the presence of mine enemies: You anoint my head with oil; my cup runs over.

*6) Surely goodness and mercy shall follow me all the days of my life: and I will dwell in the house of the L*ord *forever.*

Psalm 51

1) Have mercy upon me, O God, according to your lovingkindness: according to the multitude of your tender mercies blot out my transgressions.

2) Wash me thoroughly from my iniquity, and cleanse me from my sin.

3) For I acknowledge my transgressions: and my sin is always before me.

4) Against you, you only, have I sinned, and done this evil in your sight: that you may be just when you speak and blameless when you judge.

5) Behold, I was brought forth in iniquity, and in sin my mother conceived me.

6) Behold, You desire truth in the inward parts, and in the hidden part You will make me to know wisdom.

7) Purge me with hyssop, and I shall be clean; wash me, and I shall be whiter than snow.

8) Make me hear joy and gladness, that the bones You have broken may rejoice.

9) Hide Your face from my sins and blot out all my iniquities.

10) Create in me a clean heart, O God, and renew a steadfast spirit within me.

11) Do not cast me away from Your presence, and do not take Your Holy Spirit from me.

12) *Restore to me the joy of Your salvation, and uphold me by Your generous Spirit*

13) *Then I will teach transgressors Your ways, and sinners shall be converted to You.*

14) *Deliver me from the guilt of bloodshed, O God, the God of my salvation, and my tongue shall sing aloud of Your righteousness.*

15) *O LORD, open my lips, and my mouth shall show forth Your praise.*

16) *For You do not desire sacrifice, or else I would give it. You do not delight in burnt offering.*

17) *The sacrifices of God are a broken spirit, a broken and a contrite heart— these, O God, You will not despise.*

18) *Do good in Your good pleasure to Zion; build the wall of Jerusalem.*

19) *Then You shall be pleased with the sacrifices of righteousness, with burnt offering and whole burnt offering: then they shall offer bulls on Your altar.*

David's Prayer:
Acknowledge - Confess - Repent

David was a man of prayer. When he needed help in a given situation he was quick to call on the LORD. But prayer is more than just asking God to do things for us.

Prayer is also asking God for His forgiveness and seeking His wisdom to know what we should do to undo hurts and make things right.

There are three things David demonstrated by his actions, after being confronted by the prophet Nathan.

First David recognized and confessed his wrong doing .He was admitting he was the one responsible for his actions. David had no one else to blame. Not even the woman who had been his partner in the sexual affair.

Secondly, David repented. More than being sorry for wrong doing or feeling sorry for getting caught in a wicked act, repentance involves changing of the mind.

It is saying *"I know what I did was wrong and I now want to do the right thing. I choose to change my mind."*

The third element involves forsaking a wrong life style or action. In Psalm 101: 2-3 David said it well: *"I will walk within my house with a perfect heart. I will set no wicked things before my eyes."*

"Forsaking" is being willing to change the environment. If necessary, it could even mean giving up an undesirable relationship. It is letting go of the past and letting God do what only He can do.

God's Response
Forgive - Create - Renew

The Bible gives us simple instructions on how to deal with sin in our lives. Here is a direct quote: *"If we confess our sins, He is faithful and just to forgive us our sins and to cleanse us from all unrighteousness."*

"If we walk in the light as He is in the light, we have fellowship with one another, and the blood of Jesus Christ His Son cleanses us from all sin." (1 John 1: 9 & 7)

63

Only God can truly forgive sin. The good news is there is no sin that is too big, too bad or too ugly for God to forgive. The blood of Jesus paid the penalty for every sin.

David had a list of wrongs, maybe longer than most of us. He was guilty of both immorality and the indirect murder of the man whose wife he had taken.

God offers us the gift of a clean heart. A clean heart is one that is free from all condemnation. Having received God's forgiveness is evidenced by a clear conscience.

Keeping our hearts clean and our minds renewed, is a daily process. We have to be selective in what you think.

On a moment by moment basis, we decide what we are going to think about. Clean thoughts produce a clean mind. The blood of Jesus cleanses from all sin.

The Power of God's Word

In our daily life, we are bombarded with images and ideas that can seem to be almost irresistible. Overcoming those evil thoughts and the wicked temptations of the flesh takes supernatural power.

The good news is that we do not have to overcome evil by ourselves. 1 John 4:4 tells us *"Greater is He, [Jesus] who is in you, than he (the wicked one) who is in the world."*

John 1:12 says, *"As many as received Him [Jesus] to them gave He the power to become the sons of God."*

When we make the decision to do what is right, God gives us the power to bring it to pass. He knows that we are human and need His help.

God's will for us is only good, but He has left the choice of what we are going to do up to us and the choices we make are determined by our thoughts and desires.

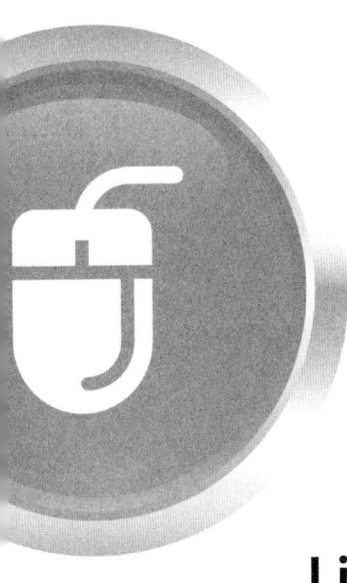

Life in the Fast Lane

Like the lurid events in the lives of King David and Bathsheba recorded in the Old Testament of the Scriptures, there is a parallel story in the New Testament.

It is the narrative of a young man who made the wrong decisions. He got into wrong company, he did wrong things, and finally ended up in the "Pigpen" of life.

It is found in the Gospel of Luke, chapter 15, and Jesus Himself, is the story teller.

Jesus began the story by saying, "A father had two sons. One day the younger of the two brothers came to his father with a request.

66

Wanting to leave the sheltered life of a farm boy, he asked the father to divide the family inheritance between him and his brother. He wanted to have his portion now."

No doubt, there was much discussion about what the younger son was asking the father to do. But realizing the determination of the young son, the father divided the family estate, giving both of his sons the portion that would ultimately become their rightful inheritance.

As a member of the traditional Jewish community, it was the custom for the older son to receive a double portion of the family inheritance. With this extra share of the estate also came the responsibility of caring for the parents in their old age.

As the story continues, it says that after not many days the younger son left and headed out to seek the thrills of life. While there are no details of his wild and unbecoming behavior mentioned, the story leads us to believe that he was an irresponsible thrill seeker with loose morals.

With a pocket full of money, he soon had lots of friends. For awhile the young man must have thought that he had the world by the tail. Still, as he was spending the money, he had inherited from his father, his conscience may have reminded him of the godly principles he had been taught as a child.

With the younger (and perhaps more aggressive) son out of the house, things may have seemed quiet on the father's farm. There likely were days when the father asked himself questions about what went wrong in the upbringing of his younger son and what he could have done differently.

Both sons had been exposed to the same counsel and teaching. Why did the younger son choose to leave? Like any caring father with a spiritual understanding, surely the father prayed for the safety of his son. More importantly, the father believed one day his prayer would be answered and the son would return.

Looking on the bright side, perhaps the father thought his son might have invested some of his assets in a business venture. Maybe he got married and one day would return with a wife. Who knows, there could even be grandchildren. But that was not to be the case.

Celebrations did not come often in the life of a farmer but when the time for celebration came, it was always a big event. According to their Jewish way of life, festivities could last for days. To be prepared for such special events, it was the custom to have a fatted calf ready as a source of fresh meat for a celebration occasion.

As we will see, things had not gone well for the younger son. His poor choice of friends and his lifestyle were draining his cash reserves. The life he had been living was too expensive for him and one day, to his dismay, he realized his money was all gone. He was flat broke!

Having established his new relationships, he thought surely now that he was in need of help, they would be there for him. But he quickly discovered that his circle of friends had only been there to help exploit the resources he had brought when he came from the farm.

He had been a poor judge of character and now his friends were nowhere in sight. He realized that he had not handled his money wisely but there was still something he could do. Having been raised on the farm, he did know how to work hard so he began looking for a job.

It seemed that circumstances of life were turning against him at every corner. A famine broke out in the country and jobs were hard to find. As unthinkable as it might have seemed, out of sheer desperation, he entered into a working relationship with someone who made his living raising hogs.

How could a Jewish boy, who understood the dietary laws of his faith, stoop so low? Hogs were considered unclean. Even touching a hog was considered a violation of good hygiene. Now he found himself in physical daily contact with these filthy creatures he had learned to despise.

History records that under Alexander the Great, and as part of the Greek culture, sometimes swine were used for their religious temple sacrifices.

Instead of a perfect lamb, a dirty pig was placed on the altar in the temple of God. This had to be a profane experience for a religious Jew to witness.

The hog partnership business did not do well and the weather did not cooperate. As the famine continued, the hog business was not good and food became scarce.

Just to survive, the young man tried to eat the very husks that the swine were eating. It was at this low point in his life, the young man came to his senses. "How low have I stooped?" Must have been his most agonizing question.

As he began thinking about his father and his home, he recalled only the good things from his past. He thought of a warm home, clean clothes and lots of food to eat. Now even the strictness of his father's ways were forgotten.

The long work hours on the farm seemed only a blur in his mind. What he really remembered was his father's goodness and the abundance his father had accumulated through his diligent and honest efforts.

On the farm, even if there hadn't been much rain, things always seemed to work out. Never in all his days had he seen even a servant go without food, warm clothing, and shelter. It would be tough and humbling to admit the error of his ways, but he knew it was time to head back home and face whatever he would have to face.

Beginning the journey home, he came to a full recognition of what he had done. He had sinned against his father as well as violated the law of God. He knew at this time there was no way he could make restitution. All he could do was to ask for forgiveness and he was willing to do it.

Realizing he had wasted his inheritance, he knew he had no more legal rights as a son but that did not matter to him anymore. He would become a servant on his father's farm if that's what it would take. If he couldn't stay in the house, he would sleep with the other hired hands.

At least he would have warm clothes, a roof over his head, and plenty to eat. He knew his father could be tough, but he also knew the goodness of the man he was about to meet. As he came closer to what was once his home, he could see the buildings now coming into view. He had made it back!

Looking up, he saw someone standing at the head of the path leading up to the house. Suddenly he saw a man running toward him. It was his father!

Likely, he had been on that path many times before waiting for the return of his son. Now it had happened! His prayers had been answered.

As the two met, the son tried to blurt out the confession of wrong doing he had memorized. Before he could finish, he was overwhelmed by the love of his father.

Looking at the disgraced image of his son, the father saw the dirty robe the son was wearing was nothing but rags and there were no shoes on his feet.

Even the ring that had been on his hand when he first left home was gone. *"Bring a new robe and a new pair of shoes, and don't forget the family ring for his hand,"* were the father's orders to his servants.

This all seemed too good to be true! Surely he did not deserve this kind of a home coming reception. All that the son had asked for was the role of a servant.

No doubt the young man who had spent time with pigs, had also acquired their odor. Before putting on the new robe and shoes he obviously took a bath.

How good it was to once again experience the love and the provision of his generous, loving, and forgiving father.

The good news that the Prodigal Son had returned spread quickly. Family, friends and neighbors were invited to a great home coming celebration.

The fatted calf, reserved for such a time as this was going to be butchered. Soon it would be time to enjoy scrumptious food and begin a time of rejoicing. With musicians in place, now it was time for the party to begin.

The father's theme for the party was, *"My son who was lost has been found. My son who was dead has come back to life."* What a joy it was for both father and son to be back together again as a happy family.

But already there were negative consequences. His older brother refused to accept him. Unforgiving, he accused the father of poor judgment.

Would he ever go back to a life in the pigpen? Never! Would he ever again doubt the goodness of his father? Absolutely not! Would he ever again question the love of his father? How could he, after all that his father had done for him by taking him back into the family?

The spiritual message told by this moving story is the faithfulness of God to forgive us even when we have no way of making restitution for wrong doing.

Did the father know the son had done wrong? Sure he did. But he also recognized that his son knew it too. That was all that really mattered.

Were there other consequences for the bad behavior of the younger son? Most likely there were. At the time of the father's death, would there be another inheritance check for him? Not likely.

There is no sin too big or too bad for God to forgive. Even after receiving forgiveness, however, some wrong actions can carry heavy consequences.

This is especially true of things that are related to illicit sexual behavior. Included in this are sexually transmitted diseases and broken relationships.

73

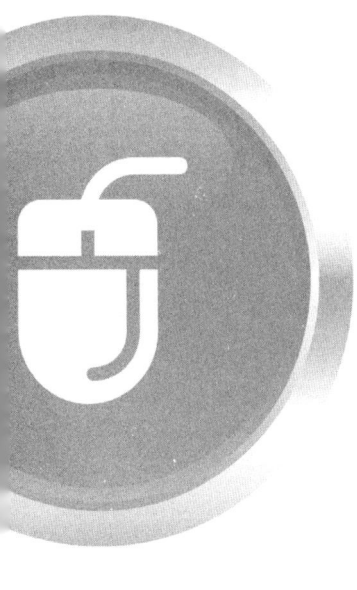

Fast Forward
3000 years

From the Time of David
into the 21st Century

Like King David's experience on the housetop, the sight of a bathing beauty is still alluring. Desire out of control is still deadly, the cost of immoral behavior still has a high price, and the unchanging law of sowing and reaping is still in effect.

The big difference between David's world and our world is that he had only one *"Bathsheba channel"* available. Today via the internet there are literally millions of pornographic web sites just a mouse click away in every online household.

Nathan, the prophet, described David's sin as something that had happened in secret when no one else was looking. So too today, there is immoral sexual enticement available online in the privacy of a bedroom, an office, or on a laptop computer.

The brain is accessed by all five of the human senses. Most rapidly and most powerfully, this happens through our eyes. In a millisecond, sexual images transmitted to the brain can begin to trigger sexual arousal and desire.

Not only is there an endless stream of sexual internet web sites available today, the content is beyond what anyone in generations past could ever have imagined. Raw sex acts, and images of sexual perversion are lurking on the web, waiting to release their deadly poison into the minds of potential victims. They are just one mouse click away.

In some areas of society today, pornography is looked at as a victimless crime. But even a shallow understanding of how the human brain works dispels this promoted misconception that pornography is a harmless and acceptable behavior.

Labeling pornography as a victimless crime is also ignoring the addictive power of porn. Like a drug in the blood stream, porn images in the mind have a similar effect to that of drug addiction. The power of addiction draws the victim back for repeated encounters.

My Personal Experience

It was in the month of March, in 1992, when I found myself stormed in at the Pittsburgh, Pennsylvania, airport. Earlier that day, I had been a guest on a Christian TV program to talk about and promote our **Wiser Family** Bible Story Videos.

We had a late blizzard and all flights were canceled so I had to spend the night in a motel nearby. Sitting alone in my motel room late that afternoon, I turned on the TV. It was set on a movie channel and I quickly realized an "R" rated movie was playing.

This was not normal behavior on my part, but using boredom as an excuse, I watched the movie anyway. There were only a few brief scenes of nudity, but as I was watching, it seemed as if something leaped from the television screen and lodged itself in my mind.

When I got back to Tulsa, I told my wife Dorothy, about my experience. We prayed together and I asked God for His forgiveness.

While I knew that God had forgiven me, those immoral scenes were still etched in my mind and I could not shake them. Too embarrassed to ask anyone for help, I fought this sexual harassment demon by myself for weeks.

I did not become immoral in my behavior and continued to minister and teach; however, even while instructing others, those suggestive movie scenes would try to replay in my mind.

Out of desperation, at the beginning of each day I began praying the prayer of David in Psalm 51:10 *"Create in me a clean heart, and renew a right spirit within me."*

I added another powerful Scripture from Psalm 101:2-3: *"I will walk within my house with a perfect heart. I will set no wicked thing before my eyes."*

I do not recall the exact moment that it happened but one morning while I was praying, I realized that the oppression was gone!

My mind had been cleansed and washed by the water of God's Word. Once again I felt like a free man.

Using the *"Sword of the Spirit,"* the demon of sexual harassment had been defeated. I knew that I had defeated the enemy in my thought life.

To this day, I still quote those same scriptures. The Word of God is the power of **The Clean Heart Prayer.** Quoting the scriptures to overcome temptation is also what Jesus did when He was tempted by the Devil.

I realize that by today's standards, many will consider this to be a trivial experience, but it taught me the importance of guarding the mind and what I allow my eyes to see.

As a father and now a grandfather, I am concerned about our children and grandchildren. I want to do what I can to help them make the right moral decisions as well.

79

Pornography Is Immoral

Pornography as well as porn web sites thrive on images and acts that are both indecent and immoral. Watching immoral behavior draws the viewer into the very immoral act emotionally and mentally.

In the words of Jesus in Matthew 5:28, when addressing issues of morality, He said, *"Whoever looks on a woman to lust for her has already committed adultery with her in his heart."*

Obviously, the same spiritual truth applies to a woman looking lustfully at a man.

Porn Sites Are Degrading

Willingly or unwillingly, individuals who are participants in the actual creation of porn are asked to do what is dirty and morally degrading. What happens in the porn industry is well known. It is vulgar, grossly exaggerated and unnecessary to describe.

The Penalty of Internet Porn

A dirty conscience, infidelity, divorce, loss of position, loss of property, loss of reputation and the destruction of families are just some of the deadly effects of addiction to internet porn. What a high price to pay for momentary sexual excitement and pleasure!

Politicians have resigned their positions and pastors have given up churches because of porn activity. Often, individuals charged with heinous sexual crimes have first been involved in some form of pornography.

While there are many and various causes of sexually transmitted diseases, internet porn is certainly a major contributing behavioral factor.

Feeding the mind on the content of porn sites can develop both natural and unnatural sexual desires. This behavior can lead to illicit physical sexual relationships, and is also the breeding ground for many related sexually transmitted diseases.

Porn Addiction Can Affect Anyone

No living human being is ever immune to sexual temptation. Today, even small children who are using the internet for study purposes can accidentally stumble across porn sites.

This also includes adults who are inexperienced with internet use. Just clicking a forwarded e-mail link can lead to an unsuspected porn site.

We have all heard or read about teenagers, young adults, married couples, senior citizens and even pastors who have found themselves with an addiction they hate to admit. That addiction is to internet pornography.

Dr. Chuck Swindoll, the *Insight for Living* radio host, in an online open letter to churches addressed the problem of internet porn in the church today. Here is his quote:

"The most recent studies available suggest that as many one out of every two people-that's 50% of the people sitting in our pews, are looking at and/or could be addicted to Internet pornography."

The problem of internet pornography is so huge that recently numerous secular media personalities have spoken out publicly about it. The dangers of this growing epidemic is sweeping the country, destroying families, marriages, and lives in its path.

Porn Addiction Can Seem Hopeless

There may be temporary pleasure in watching porn but for every minute of pleasure there are hours of guilt.

It is not uncommon to hear about a porn addict traveling across the country, spending days and thousands of dollars to meet someone for just momentary, illicit sexual stimulation and gratification.

Hating themselves for what they are doing and realizing the evil of their ways, many still find it impossible to change their undesirable behavior.

Too embarrassed to ask for help, they struggle alone. Self condemnation, broken resolutions and failure after failure, causing a sense of despair.

Feelings of hopelessness and low self worth come from the repeated unsuccessful attempts to end this addictive negative and hated behavior.

Understanding the spiritual side of addiction, helps to shed light on why change is so difficult or even impossible, when the attempt is purely in the area of the mind.

There are spiritual wicked forces at work that attack the mind. Breaking loose from evil forces takes more than will power; it takes the power of the Word of God.

In John 8:32, Jesus said, that when we know the truth, the truth would also set us free.

Jesus, the Son of God, demonstrated this when He was tempted by the wicked one in the wilderness. Repeatedly He used the words of scripture as the ultimate weapon against temptation.

That is why the scriptures tell us to use the Sword of the Spirit and the Shield of Faith as our weapons against the evil attacks of the Devil.

The Best Answer Is Stop before You Start

The best answer to the pornography problem is to stop before you start. Porn addiction begins in the mind so keep the mind pure.

Here is both the question and the answer taken from the Scriptures in Psalm 119:9: "How can a young man keep his way pure? By living according to your Word."

83

Of course the same admonition also applies to a young woman. A sure way to keep the mind clean is to renew it daily with scriptures from God's Word because there is power in God's Word.

Hebrews 4:12 says, *"The Word of God is quick (Alive) and powerful, and it is sharper than a two-edged sword."(KJV)*

Here is a direct quote taken from the sixth chapter in the book of Deuteronomy. It was a prayer called the Shema, prayed twice daily by a Jewish family.

This was God's instruction given through Moses to each family in Israel, in Deuteronomy, chapter 6:

> *4 Hear, O Israel: The Lord our God, the Lord is one!*
> *5 You shall love the Lord your God with all your heart, with all your soul, and with all your strength.*
> *6 And these words which I command you today shall be in your heart.*
> *7 You shall teach them diligently to your children, and shall talk of them when you sit in your house, when you walk by the way, when you lie down, and when you rise up.*
> *8 You shall bind them as a sign on your hand, and they shall be as frontlets between your eyes.*
> *9 You shall write them on the doorposts of your house and on your gates."*

These instructions that were spoken by the voice of God are still applicable today. Our Creator, who formed the human mind, knows how it operates. That is why we are told to renew the mind daily.

Psalm 1 offers these added words of instruction:

> *1 Blessed is the man who walks not in the counsel of the ungodly, nor stands in the path of sinners, nor sits in the seat of the scornful;*
> *2 But his delight is in the law of the LORD, and in His law he meditates day and night.*
> *3 He shall be like a tree planted by the rivers of water, that brings forth its fruit in its season, whose leaf*

also shall not wither; and whatever he does shall prosper.

4 *The ungodly are not so, but are like the chaff which the wind drives away.*

5 *Therefore the ungodly shall not stand in the judgment, Nor sinners in the congregation of the righteous.*

6 *For the LORD knows the way of the righteous, but the way of the ungodly shall perish.*

85

WHAT DO YOU THINK?

I guard my mind and what I think.
Thoughts are seeds that grow.
I meditate on what is true,
And I reap what I sow.

The sites online, the books I read,
The movies and TV,
Are painting pictures in my mind,
Of what I think and see.

I do not do this by myself.
I found a better way.
I talk to God and ask for help,
As I start each new day.

© Peter Enns 2011

THE CLEAN HEART PRAYER!

"Create in me a clean heart, O God; and
renew a right spirit within me". (Psalm 51:10)

"Let the words of my mouth, and the
meditation of my heart, be acceptable
in your sight, O Lord". (Psalm 19:14)

"Your word have I hid in my heart, that
I might not sin against thee". (Psalm 119:11 NKJV)

"I will walk within my house with a
perfect heart. I will set nothing wicked
before my eyes;" (Psalm. 101:2-3 NKJV)

"As for me and my house, we will
serve the Lord". (Joshua 24:15)

GO BACK HOME
THE FATHER IS WAITING!

Leaving his home, he went out to enjoy,
The things he had missed, as a sheltered farm boy.
The glitz and the glamour! The sounds and the sights!
He had pleasure filled days and passion filled nights.

Forgetting his morals, his mind filled with trash,
He had lots of friends, till he ran out of cash.
How quickly things changed. He was looking for work.
Living with hogs, he felt like a jerk.

In the pigpen of life, a heart filled with shame!
He came to himself. He had no one to blame.
The good life was gone. Now sitting in lack.
The prodigal son said, "I'm going back."

Since the day that he left, the father had prayed,
That God would bring back the son who had strayed.
There was joy in the house! The son had returned.
Forgiven by God. What a lesson he'd learned.

© Peter Enns 2011

88

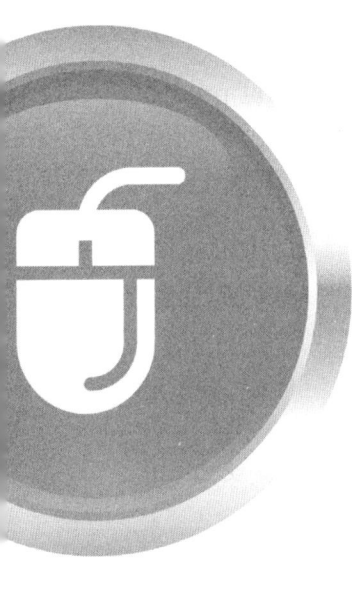

S.T.O.P.
Straight Talk On
Pornography

Digital Prodigals

Today we are living in a world of digital prodigals. No longer is it necessary to travel to a far country to indulge in and enjoy sensual illicit pleasures. The far country is all around us, and just an online internet mouse click away.

Digital prodigals come in all sizes and all colors. They are the young and the old, they are male and female. They include both professionals and common laborers. They are the powerful and the weak; there are no exceptions.

They even include pastors and those in church leadership. What they each have in common is a life in the pigpen and likely, they hate what they have become.

Certainly it did not start that way. At first it was only a look of curiosity. What's out there that I have not seen? But then it began to progress.

Going back to the same online web site, there were links to other related sites. An appetite for erotic images began to develop and a terrible addiction began.

The resulting sexual images in the mind become a source of gratification that is neither good nor wholesome. The isolation of being alone on the computer has become a way of life. Time spent at erotic online sites becomes a blur as the hours slip away.

Even away from the screen, the mind continues to replay immoral scenes that have been mentally recorded. What began as a casual look now has turned into an obsession. Ashamed of what is happening and too embarrassed to ask for help, the tracks now have to be covered. But sooner or later, someone, somewhere, will find out.

Loaded with guilt, the digital prodigal is longing to go back to the days of a clean mind and a clear conscience. Repeatedly there are resolutions to stop this destructive behavior but with each temptation they are also quickly abandoned and broken.

Life for the digital prodigal has become like a theme park. There are highs and there are lows, including moments of excitement. But mostly, it seems that life is just going in circles. Like a person on a tread mill, they are making an effort but seem to be getting nowhere.

So how does the digital prodigal get out of this downward spiral and come back to having a clean heart and a renewed mind, even in a dirty world?

The answer is the same as it was for King David and his affair with Bathsheba, and the story of the Prodigal Son. You have to make the decision to stop. If you don't; it is going to stop you.

Voluntarily or involuntarily, one day the Digital Prodigal will be discovered. Whether it be the young man in the fast lane of life, the lusting pastor in the pulpit, the bored housewife surfing the internet, or the perverted politician sending lurid e-mail. Sooner or later, the sad day of discovery is coming for each of them.

Here are two important scriptures the Digital Prodigal needs to remember. They are Numbers 32:23, *"Be sure your sin will find you out,"* and Proverbs 28:13 *"He who covers his sins shall not prosper. But he who confesses and forsakes shall find mercy."*

STOP really means coming to the end of oneself and his or her own ways. Neither King David nor the Prodigal Son stopped their wrongful behavior until they had run out of all options. For David, it ended with the murder of Uriah. For the Prodigal Son, it was running out of money and finding himself in the pigpen.

STOP means that I am willing to accept responsibility for all my decisions and corresponding actions. While there may have been other contributors involved, I was the decision maker. It is David's prayer for forgiveness and the Prodigal saying "Father, I have sinned and I am so sorry."

STOP is also recognizing that I have gone the wrong way. I am out of resources and I cannot get out of this pigpen by myself. It is making a decision and taking the first step in the direction of home. It is trusting in God's grace and relying on His mercy and His ability to restore the fallen.

STOP is more than getting caught in the act. It is a heart of true repentance. It is sorrow for the pain and hurt that negative actions may have caused. But repentance is more than an emotion. Repentance is having a change of mind and then going in a new direction.

STOP includes acknowledging the goodness of God. Like the return of the Prodigal Son, there is joy and rejoicing when a Digital Prodigal makes the decision to return home. It is receiving and putting on a clean robe, and burning the old dirty rags. It includes new shoes to go in a new direction.

STOP is accepting the family ring and realizing that the Father still trusts me and once more, I am part of the family. The ring is the symbol of the family status in the community as well as a token of delegated authority.

It may take time, but the Father will give me a new assignment. Knowing the hard lessons that we have learned from our bad experiences makes us more valuable and qualified to take on the new tasks the Father may have for us.

STOP is renewing the mind daily with scriptures from the Bible. Becoming a Digital Prodigal was more than looking at explicit images.

There were negative spiritual forces at work as well, seeking to kill and destroy.

STOP could mean you need to clean up your computer hard drive. There may be images imbedded on the system you are not aware of. Like the dirty rags of the Prodigal Son, they need to be removed and destroyed.

STOP could also be adding an internet content filter to your computer. Their are a variety of content filters available online. **Blue Coat Systems** offers an excellent **Free Content Filter**.

The content filter can be downloaded at **"No Charge"** and set to block everything from hate speech to violence as well as sites with explicit sexual content.

Blue Coat Systems Inc. (www.bluecoat.com) has also granted a license to **Good Word Publishing** to help promote the content filter. www1.k9webprotection.com

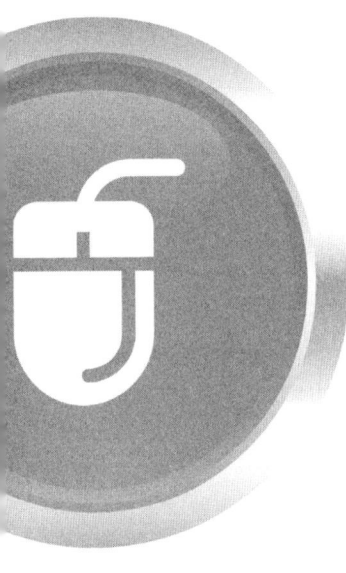

S.T.A.R.T.
Straight Talk About
Right Thinking

START AGAIN

Make a new beginning,
And leave the past behind.
God has a plan for winning,
Let truth renew your mind.

Your life is what you make it,
And you set your own worth.
The prize is yours, so take it,
It's yours by right of birth.

Trust God for direction.
To walk by faith you must.
You'll have divine protection,
When in God you trust.

© Peter Enns 2011

Making a New Beginning

Y ou want to make a new beginning? That's good! So where do you start? The best place to begin is in the beginning. Genesis 1:1 says, *"In the beginning God created the heavens and the earth."*

Throughout the entire creation process we are reminded of the goodness of God by the repeated statement God made, when He said, *"It is good!"*

God started the human experience on the earth by creating one man and one woman. When God looked at the two humans He had made, He said, *"It is very good!"* God put them in charge and gave them authority to rule and have dominion over every other creation on earth.

As surely as God is good, there is another force that is evil. Add a D to evil and you have it. It is the Devil! God and the Devil are total opposites. Opposites, but definitely not equals! God is only good and the Devil is only bad.

God is light the Devil is darkness. God creates life and the Devil destroys life. God's Word is truth and the Devil is a liar. God loves and the Devil hates. God blesses; the Devil curses.

As humans, we have the choice of whom we will serve. The first temptation started with a suggestion from the evil one that God could not be trusted. The Devil implied there

97

was something God did not want Adam and Eve to know. At that critical moment, the first woman on earth, made the decision to doubt what God had said.

Eve chose to believe the words of the Devil. With her husband Adam in full agreement, they both ate of the forbidden fruit, breaking the commandment of God. In theological terms, this resulted in "The Fall of Man."

Evil had made its way into man's world. God had created mankind with a free will and mankind had chosen to walk in disobedience. Their decision separated mankind from the intimate relationship they had with God.

But God still loved mankind and had a plan. One day He would send a Savior who would come to earth to reunite mankind with God through His plan of salvation.

From the day of his creation until today, mankind has had the opportunity of choice. In Deuteronomy, chapter 28, God's Word says, *"I set before you life and death, blessing and cursing."* To make it easy, God's Word says, *"Choose life!"*

As illustrated in the life of King David, good people still have the freedom to make bad choices. God had called David, *"A man after His own heart."*

Still, this man who was anointed by God to be the next great King of Israel, by his own decision ended up in the "Pigpen," of life. But then, heeding the Word of the Prophet Nathan, David made a new beginning.

David's prayer for God to *"Create in me a clean heart and renew a right spirit within me,"* was heard and answered by God. To add glory to the story, God allowed David to be in the ancestral line of Jesus, who would one day be born of the Virgin Mary.

God, who is perfect, all wise, and all powerful, for His own reason, made the decision to give us an example of what it means to start again. Adam, created by God, and called the son of God, through his disobedience had caused the sinful fall of the human race.

Now God was starting again with another person, also called the Son of God. Born of the Virgin Mary, He was God's only begotten Son, meaning He was the only Son who was born of a woman. His name was Jesus. Eve had doubted God's Word but Mary chose to believe it!

Jesus came to this earth to pay for the penalty of sin for the entire human race. But in the interim, between His birth and His death, He also showed us the character of God. To the Old Testament believers, God was the Almighty Creator. But Jesus revealed God to us as a loving Father.

In the parable of the Prodigal Son as well as in the LORD's Prayer, Jesus talked about God as a loving, caring Heavenly Father. God saw the human race in the pigpen

99

of life, dirty and undeserving. Then He made a way for each of us to come back home and become part of His wonderful family again.

To God, starting over was entering into a New Covenant with mankind. Beginning with Abraham, the Old Covenant had lasted until the death of Jesus. During the Last Supper, Jesus foreshadowed the coming of the New Covenant. The wine in the cup symbolized the blood He would shed as His part in it.

Just a few days later in the Garden of Gethsemane, Jesus, the sinless Son of God took upon Himself the sins of the entire human race. He was offering Himself as the final sacrifice, as the spotless Lamb of God.

He was taking on the sins of the whole world. The scriptures say that the task was so difficult that under the pressure of it, literal drops of blood came out of His perspiration pores.

Hanging on a cruel cross, falsely accused, Jesus, the Son of God died, not for any wrong that He had done; but rather, Jesus was dying as a sacrificial Lamb. Prophesied by John the Baptist, Jesus had come as the Lamb of God to take away the sins of the world.

Abandoned by the very God of Creation, Jesus cried out, *"My God, My God, why have you forsaken Me!"* At that very moment, the Old Covenant was finished. When Jesus shouted the words, *"It is finished!"* He was also saying that the price of the penalty for the sins of mankind; past, present and future had been paid.

The final words of Jesus on the cross, *"Father, into Your hands I commend My spirit,"* was the beginning of a new relationship between God and mankind. It was the start of a new family relationship between a loving Father and His estranged children.

The price for the penalty of sin had been paid and the Old Covenant was finished. Now a New Covenant was established but there was still one more enemy that had to be defeated. It was the enemy of death, the ultimate consequence of sin. God was making a totally new beginning for mankind.

101

Jesus had died and paid for the penalty of sin and defeated death itself. Now He was being raised from the dead. As the power of God began to surge into His lifeless body in the grave, Jesus became the firstborn of the dead. Jesus had conquered both sin and death. The grave could not hold Him. Jesus was alive for evermore!

Only fifty days after His resurrection, Jesus and a select group of His followers met on the Mount of Olives.

After giving them His final instructions, something very amazing happened. Gravity lost its grip on Jesus and He began to rise into the sky.

Those who were there with Him watched in wonder as they saw Him ascend, till He disappeared into the clouds. Suddenly two angelic beings appeared with this message: they said, *"Just as you have seen Him go away, Jesus will return one day."*

The world today is very weary of bad news. Talk about terror, war, earthquakes and famines can leave us feeling helpless and hopeless. But the promise of the Second Coming of Jesus in Acts 1:11, is good news. It is part of the Gospel message.

Being ready for the return of Jesus, is not based on any religious or moral code. It is based on a relationship. Believing that Jesus, born of a virgin, came as the Lamb of God to die for the penalty of sin for mankind, is the basis of our faith.

Our relationship with God begins by being "Born Again!" A common term used in evangelical circles; what does it really mean to be "Born Again?"

Birth always follows conception. To be "Born Again," is a personal and a spiritual experience. It begins with our Father in heaven and results in us becoming a part of His family, by faith in His Word.

Hearing God's Word and believing the message of salvation by faith, in the finished work of Jesus, is like spiritual conception. That is when spiritual life begins.

102

Here is how the apostle Paul explains being "Born Again," in Romans Chapter 10 Verses 9 & 10.

"If you confess with your mouth the Lord Jesus and believe in your heart that God has raised Him from the dead, you will be saved. For with the heart one believes unto righteousness, and with the mouth confession is made unto salvation."

Our faith is activated when we confess our belief in Jesus, the LAMB OF GOD, dying on the cross. By an act of our will we acknowledge that we were under the penalty of sin, but Jesus paid the price for our salvation.

When God raised Jesus from the dead, the salvation process was completed. Jesus was given a Name which is above every other name. Jesus is LORD!

103

If you have never done it before, or if you are unsure of your relationship with God, this is your personal opportunity to be "Born Again." Say it in your own words, or use this prayer as a guideline. Speak it out so you can hear yourself.

"Father, I come to You at Your invitation and in the Name of Your Son, Jesus. I recognize that as part of the human race, I too am a sinner, both by my inheritance and by my own actions. I understand that the wages of sin is death.

I believe Jesus, Your Son, came to earth and by His death He paid for the penalty for the sins of mankind, including my sin and my wrong doing. I believe that You raised Him from the dead and that He is alive today.

I believe that all power has been given to Him by You and Jesus is LORD! I now accept Jesus as my Savior and You as my Father. Thank you for Your love and the wonderful plan You have for me. Amen."

Being "Born Again," we are members of God's family. We are His sons and daughters and Jesus is now our older brother. The Bible says we are joint heirs with Jesus.

Because of His relationship with God, His Father, Jesus extends a special privilege to the other family members as well. When we pray to our Father, we can come to Him in "Jesus' Name."

It is like Jesus giving us His "Power of Attorney" to use whenever we pray. What an awesome privilege this is, and what a great God we serve!

PUBLIC AUCTION

Mankind was on the auction block.
The bidding price was high.
Without another bidder,
Mankind would have to die.

God was mankind's maker.
Mankind had lost his way.
And wasted heaven's treasure.
With nothing left to pay.

God knew this day was coming.
He had a secret plan,
Hanging on a rugged cross,
He paid the price for man.

The price kept going higher.
God turned and hid His face.
His son, condemned, forsaken,
Was taking mankind's place.

When He cried, "It is finished!"
The highest price was in.
The price had been accepted.
God's love had paid for sin.

© Peter Enns 2011

105

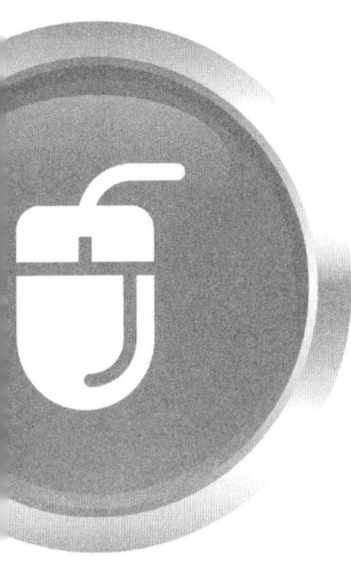

S.T.A.N.D.
Straight Talk About
New Decisions

There is a story in the Bible about King Ahab who came from a good family and married a woman named Jezebel, who came from a bad family. To this day, the name Jezebel is still used to describe a woman of low moral standards.

Jezebel was the first lady of the kingdom. Her influence and example led the nation of Israel in a downward spiral. It was at this point that the Prophet Elijah was called by God into a confrontation with King Ahab, the queen and the prophets of Baal.

1 Kings 18:21 records the challenging words of Elijah as he calls on the people to make a decision between right and wrong. *"How long will you falter between two opinions?"* is his demanding question. It was time for the nation to make up its mind and decide whom they were going to serve.

Our nation and our world today face a similar question and it is time for us to make up our minds. Will we serve the god of pleasure or the God who is our Creator? Praying **The Clean Heart Prayer!** will help us take a stand and make the right personal decision.

The Decision on Trash

We live in a health conscious world today and reading food labels is emphasized. We are told to avoid too much salt and sugar, and that is good. We need to apply the same diligence in the arena of the mind. Much of so called "entertainment" today, really should have a trash content warning label on it.

To have and maintain a healthy and clean mind, we must make the decision to avoid the deliberate intake of indecent and immoral trash.

The Decision on Trust

There is a popular saying, *"If it feels good, do it."* This is a sure recipe for disaster. We cannot afford to trust our emotions or be led by our feelings. The only sure thing we can trust, is to *"Trust in the LORD!"*

In Psalm 37:3 the psalmist wrote, *"Trust in the LORD and do good; dwell in the land, and feed on His faithfulness."*

Another companion scripture in Proverbs 3: 5 & 6 tells us to *"Trust in the LORD with all your heart, and lean not on your own understanding. In all your ways acknowledge Him, and He shall direct your paths."*

The Decision on Truth

Truth is the opposite of falsehood. God is the author of truth and the Devil is the father of lies. One of the lies of Satan is the concept that God does not want us to enjoy life, when the exact opposite is true. Like the Prodigal Son, we too can chase so called pleasure and end up in the pigpen of life.

The only sure thing today is the Word of God. The Bible says that God watches over His Word to perform it.

If God said it, we can bank on it. Things may not always happen like we think they should, but we can rest assured that the laws of God will never fail.

Jesus, Himself, made this profound statement in John 14:6, *"I am the way the truth and the life. No one comes to the Father but by Me."* Trusting God and His Word is the right decision every time.

The Decision on Triumph

Triumph is ultimate victory. Go for it! When Jesus rose from the grave He had been triumphant over all the forces of evil. They could not hold Him in death and He rose victoriously.

110

After Jesus rose from the grave, He said, *"All power is given unto Me in heaven and on earth!"* This includes dominion over Satan and his evil demonic forces. Satan is real and so is temptation, but he is not our master.

We do not have to succumb to his evil ways. The Bible says when we resist the Devil, he will literally flee from us. We can be triumphant in our battle against evil but we need to have on the whole armor of God as outlined in Ephesians 6:10-18.

Beginning with the helmet of Salvation, we have on the breastplate of Righteousness, the shield of Faith and the sword of the Spirit, which is the spoken Word of God.

Using the shield of Faith we will be able to quench every fiery dart of Satan. He is no match for the sword of the Spirit. At the same time we are still instructed to flee from the lures of temptation.

When we do battle God's way, like David when he faced the giant, we too can declare, *"The battle is the LORD's!"*

Finally, we have this promise from 1 Corinthians 10:13: *"No temptation has overtaken you except such as is common to man; but God is faithful, who will not allow you to be tempted beyond what you are able, but with the temptation will also make the way of escape, that you may be able to bear it."*

A great final scripture verse on the subject comes from 2 Corinthians 2:14: *"Now thanks be to God who always leads us in triumph in Christ."* NKJV

When we speak God's Word we are renewing our mind while we are using the Sword of the Spirit against the evil one who comes to tempt us. God's Word says we can be more than conquerors when we do things God's way.

111

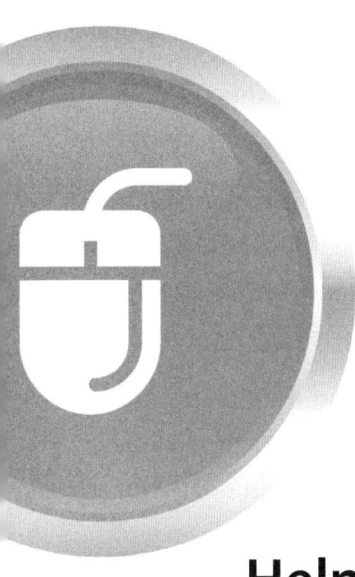

Helping Someone Else
Keep A Clean Heart

Good Godly Guidelines

I am not a psychiatrist or a psychologist trained in the cause or the cure of negative human behavior patterns.

Rather, my qualifications are being the husband of one wife for more than fifty years, resulting in three children and nine grandchildren, who (at the time of this writing) are mostly in their teens and becoming young adults.

Having lived in a strong religious community for the past forty years, I have also been involved in various church activities. This includes ten years as an instructor in a Bible Institute as well as leadership roles in several Christian businessmen's organizations.

In my experience, I have seen numerous moral failures both among lay people as well as those in leadership. This includes pastors and politicians; youth ministers and church worship leaders.

In addition, on various occasions, my wife Dorothy and I have both been asked to give counsel to couples facing morality issues in their marriages.

Some of my opinions may seem old fashioned, but so is the problem of sexual temptation. After all, the examples used in this book were all individuals who lived long ago.

Good lives and good homes are not built on popular ideas. They are built on good and Godly principles.

The alarming statistics of internet porn addiction quoted earlier in this book likely include many families where only one person is infected by this deadly plague.

No doubt, this leaves many others who may be aware of the problem but do not know what to do about it.

Protect Your Own House

The Clean Heart Prayer! is based on God's Word and every statement is personalized and individualized. This includes Psalm 101:2-3, *"I will walk within my house with a perfect heart. I will set no wicked thing before my eyes,"* and the affirmation in Joshua 24:15 *"As for me and my house, we will serve the LORD."*

Your house begins with your mind. Only you can control your own thought life. The reformer Martin Luther, said it well, "You can't stop birds from flying over your head but you can stop them from nesting in your hair."

Before you try to help someone else, realize that you too can be vulnerable. Our family physician made me aware of this. He said that as a doctor, while attending to those that are sick, he himself was constantly being exposed to germs, diseases and contagious infections.

Innocent individuals have been pulled into the addictive trap of pornography in the name of doing "Research." Curiosity and just wanting to find out what actually was "Out there," was all it took.

Several years ago, I remember reading Billy Graham's **My Answer,** newspaper column. Question: "Is it wrong for a husband and wife to watch pornography together to enhance their physical relationship."

Billy Graham's Answer: "Any marriage needing to feed on explicit sexual images is already in trouble." I agree.

The first step in helping someone else become free from the addiction of pornography is to live by your own moral values. More than porn on the internet, this also includes what you watch on television and your choice of movies at the theater.

Trust the Power of Prayer

While this may seem overly simplistic, the most powerful thing to do for the person you want to help is to pray. Specifically pray that his or her eyes will be opened to the negative effects of their addictive behavior.

Secondly, pray that the person will have the faith to believe that they can live free from the overwhelming power of porn addiction. Many individuals involved in pornography actually hate what they are doing.

They know it is wrong and time and again they have tried to quit. Because of their repeated failed attempts they have given up and now feel hopelessly bound (Not to mention the shame and the guilt they feel).

Thirdly, pray that someone who is spiritually qualified will come into their life to give them the input needed to help solve and overcome the problem.

As stated earlier in this book, lust is desire, out of control. When lust controls a person's mind, it seems all logic is lost and only the pleasure of the moment matters.

There is also an element to porn addiction that may set it apart from other addictions, including drugs or alcohol. That is a controlling spirit of lust. While sexual attraction is natural, there can also be demonic forces at play.

This is evidenced by frequent TV News stories of heinous sexually related crimes, committed by individuals who seem to be under the control of demonic forces.

Jesus said, *"All things are possible to those who believe."* This includes speaking to controlling evil forces and telling them to leave the minds of the victims they have oppressed or possessed.

Remember, as human beings each individual has a free will. Before a person can be freed from evil influences they need to desire to be free.

We cannot over-ride the will of other people. However, we can still pray that God will give them insight as well as faith to believe that they can be free from addictions and other evil influences.

117

Know Your Limitations

You can only help those individuals who want to be helped. King David, a man after God's own heart, had to come to the end of himself before God sent the prophet to speak to him. The Prodigal Son was broke and broken before he made the decision to return back to his father.

This creates a difficult situation when the person who has the addiction is a mate or a loved family member. It takes both spiritual maturity and discernment to know how to deal with these situations. While things sometimes look hopeless to us, as long as we have life, we can stand on the promises of God.

There are other good outside resources available today. They may include spiritual as well as psychological counseling. In my opinion, the most successful counseling will come from those counselors who have both spiritual as well as psychological insight into the behavior of individuals with an addiction to porn.

The Clean Heart Prayer only works when we pray it in faith. We can pray it for ourselves as well as for our loved ones. Praying God's Word, we are unleashing the most powerful force in the created universe!

In Jeremiah 1:12, God says that He watches over His Word to perform it.

A Prayer for Yourself
Based on Psalm 139:23-24

"Father, I come to You at Your invitation and in the Name of Jesus. Like David, a man after Your own heart, I too pray: "Search me, O God, and know my heart; try me, and know my thoughts; and see if there be any wicked way in me, and lead me in the way everlasting.""

Father, I know that there is nothing hidden from You. You see everything; even those things that we do in the dark. I ask for forgiveness where I have yielded to the sinful desires of my flesh. Wash my mind clean with water of Your Word.

Right now, by faith and according to Your Word, I receive Your forgiveness and cleansing from all unrighteousness.

I recognize the LORDSHIP of Jesus and I ask Him to be the LORD of my life.

Amen.

A Prayer for a Loved One

Father, I come to You at Your invitation
and in the Name of Jesus, on behalf
of: (My spouse/son/daughter/friend)

_____ .

I ask You to give (him/her) insight into
the danger and damage of exposure to
pornography.

Give: _____ a desire to have
a clean heart and a renewed mind.

I ask You to give: _____
the understanding of the power of
speaking Your Word in prayer.

Grant (him/her) the faith to believe that
with Your help, (he/she) can overcome
every temptation and be freed from any
negative addictions in (his/her) life.

Bring the right people into (his/her) life,
who will have a positive influence on:

_____ .

Lord, give me the understanding and
the wisdom to know how to best help:

_____ .

Guide me to know when to speak and when to remain silent.

I pray this prayer in faith, believing that You have heard me and that You will do what You have said You will do.

I now thank You in advance for the answer and the good things You are doing in the life of: _____ .

Amen.

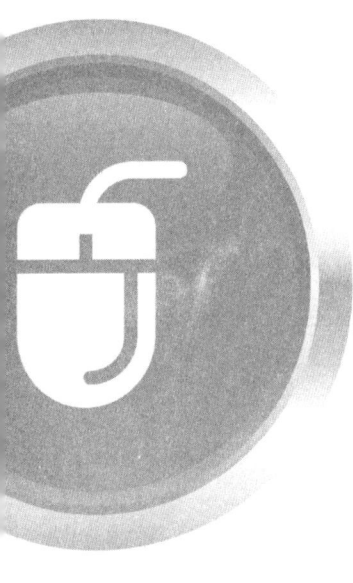

A Good Word
From the Author

THE LAWS OF GOD

You were created by God to succeed.
He purposed a place and created a need.
A need you can fill by your life day by day.
Start lending a hand to a friend on the way.

For your fondest dreams can only come true,
When you help others. They have dreams too!
By giving you get. By sowing you reap.
By serving you gain a reward you can keep.

By lending a hand to your fellowman,
You harness a law that is part of God's plan.
A law that will bring you true riches indeed,
As you set your goals in your life to succeed.

© Peter Enns 2011

MY PURPOSE

God has a purpose, just for me.
Help me Lord, so I may see,
Needs around me, I can fill.
Speak to me, while I am still.

I know your voice Lord. Here am I.
What I lack, you will supply.
With your help, I know I can,
Fulfill my purpose and your plan.

Each day I want to do my best.
Because I'm yours, I know I'm blessed.
I'm confident I will succeed.
As I work to fill a need.

© Peter Enns 2011

125

DON'T WORRY

Worry is the Devil's Trick.
It can make your body sick.
If you let it have its way,
It will steal your joy away.

Worry fills your mind with doubt,
And tells you things will not work out.
A doubting heart cannot believe.
A worried mind can not receive.

Feed your faith. Take time to pray.
Cast your cares on God each day.
Worried thoughts make you distressed.
But God is good. He wants you blessed.

© Peter Enns 2011

TOMORROW BEGINS TODAY!

Tomorrow seems uncertain, but know God has a plan.

A purpose to accomplish. If you believe, you can.

Today begins your future, don't let it slip away.

You will have tomorrow, what you believe today!

Some will say "You're dreaming. It can never be."

Stay strong and be encouraged! One day you will see.

Your words about tomorrow, helped prepare the way.

You will see tomorrow, what you say today!

Find a hurt and heal it. Today help fill a need.

The things you do for others, grow like a planted seed.

Harvest time is certain and you will get your pay.

You will reap tomorrow, what you sow today!

Today you feel rejected. Tomorrow you're a hit.

As long as there's tomorrow, tough people never quit.

If your strength is failing, take time to rest and pray.

You will be tomorrow, what you prepare today!

© Peter Enns 2011

ABOUT THE AUTHOR

On January 1, 1972, my wife Dorothy and I made the decision to create and produce **Stories That Live**; a series of children's Bible story books and audio tapes.

In 1973 we moved from Canada to Tulsa, Oklahoma. During the late 1980's, I wrote, narrated and produced a new series of **Kids International**, Bible story videos.

Cumulative product sales of our Bible story books, tapes, videos and DVDs, currently exceed three million copies.

Through the years I have been involved in various other church and ministry related activities. This includes ten years as an instructor at **Victory Bible Institute.**

In my lifetime, I have seen numerous moral failures, both among lay people as well as those in leadership. This includes pastors and politicians; evidence that no one is immune to; or exempt from sexual temptation.

While much has changed since 1972, much has also remained the same. Today's families still need a solid Biblical foundation and children still need the guidance of good parents and grandparents.

That is why I made the decision to write this book titled: **Keeping A Clean Heart in a Dirty World.**

Peter Enns

A NOTE FROM THE AUTHOR

This book is for everybody. Please read it before giving it to someone else. Let them know you have read it and how it has affected your personal life.

Good Word Publishing would like to hear from you. Constructive comments and suggestions are always welcome.

Good Word Publishing

www.mycleanheart.com